The Super Easy Air Fryer Cooking Guide

Simple & Healthy Air Fryer Dishes For Weight Loss

Ellie Sloan

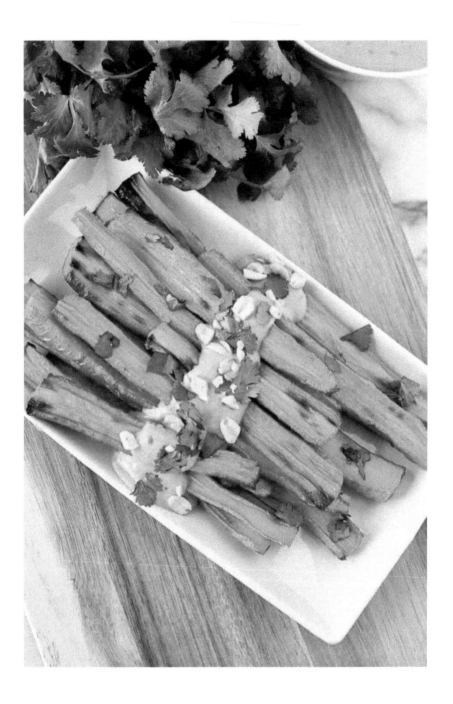

Table of contents

Baked Potatoes with Bacon

Preparation Time: 5 minutes

Cooking time: 30 minutes

Servings: 4

Ingredients:

- 4 potatoes, scrubbed, halved, cut lengthwise
- 1 tbsp. olive oil
- Salt and black pepper to taste
- 4 oz bacon, chopped

Directions

1. Preheat Air Fryer to 390°F. Brush the potatoes with olive oil and season with salt and pepper. Arrange them in the greased frying basket, cut-side down.
2. Bake for 15 minutes, flip them, top with bacon and bake for 12-15 minutes or until potatoes are golden and bacon is crispy. Serve warm.

Nutrition:

Calories 150

Fat 7g

Carbs 9g

Protein 12g

Walnut & Cheese Filled Mushrooms

Preparation Time: 5 minutes

Cooking time: 10 minutes

Servings: 4

Ingredients:

- 4 large portobello mushroom caps
- ⅓ cup walnuts, minced
- 1 tbsp. canola oil
- ½ cup mozzarella cheese, shredded
- 2 tbsp. fresh parsley, chopped

Directions

1. Preheat Air Fryer to 350°F. Grease the Air Fryer basket with cooking spray.
2. Rub the mushrooms with canola oil and fill them with mozzarella cheese. Top with minced walnuts and arrange on the bottom of the greased Air Fryer basket. Bake for 10 minutes or until golden on top. Remove, let

cool for a few minutes and sprinkle with freshly chopped parsley to serve.

Nutrition:

Calories 110

Fat 5g

Carbs 6g

Protein 8g

Air-Fried Chicken Thighs

Preparation Time: 5 minutes

Cooking time: 15 minutes

Servings: 4

Ingredients:

- 1 ½ lb. chicken thighs
- 2 eggs, lightly beaten
- 1 cup seasoned breadcrumbs
- ½ tsp. oregano
- Salt and black pepper, to taste

Directions:

1. Preheat Air Fryer to 390°F. Season the chicken with oregano, salt, and pepper. In a bowl, add the beaten eggs. In a separate bowl, add the breadcrumbs. Dip chicken thighs in the egg wash, then roll them in the breadcrumbs and press firmly so the breadcrumbs stick well.

2. Spray the chicken with cooking spray and arrange on the frying basket in a single layer, skin-side up. Air Fry for 12 minutes, turn the chicken thighs over and continue cooking for 6-8 more minutes. Serve.

Nutrition:

Calories 190

Fat 8g

Carbs 11g

Protein 16g

Simple Buttered Potatoes

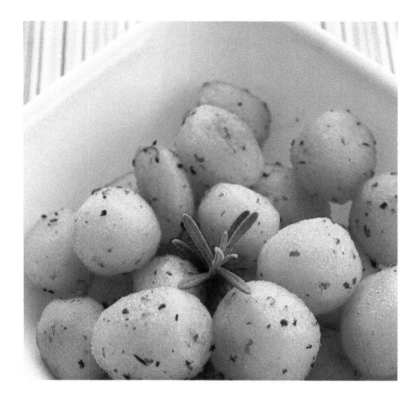

Preparation Time: 5 minutes

Cooking time: 30 minutes

Servings: 4

Ingredients:

- 1 lb. potatoes, cut into wedges
- 2 garlic cloves, grated
- 1 tsp. fennel seeds
- 2 tbsp. butter, melted
- Salt and black pepper to taste

Directions

1. In a bowl, mix the potatoes, butter, garlic, fennel seeds, salt, and black pepper, until they are well-coated. Set up the potatoes in the Air Fryer basket.
2. Bake on 360°F for 25 minutes, shaking once during cooking until crispy on the outside and tender on the inside. Serve warm.

Nutrition:

Calories 100

Fat 4g

Carbs 8g

Protein 7g

Homemade Peanut Corn Nuts

Preparation Time: 5 minutes

Cooking time: 20 minutes

Servings: 4

Ingredients:

- 6 oz dried hominy, soaked overnight
- 3 tbsp. peanut oil
- 2 tbsp. old bay seasoning
- Salt to taste

Directions

1. Preheat Air Fryer to 390°F.
2. Pat dry hominy and season with salt and old bay seasoning. Drizzle with oil and toss to coat. Spread in the Air Fryer basket and Air Fry for 10-12 minutes. Remove to shake up and return to cook for 10 more minutes until crispy. Transfer to a towel-lined plate to soak up the excess fat. Let cool and serve.

Nutrition:

Calories 100

Fat 3g

Carbs 3g

Protein 5g

Duck Fat Roasted Red Potatoes

Preparation Time: 5 minutes

Cooking time: 25 minutes

Servings: 4

Ingredients:

- 4 red potatoes, cut into wedges
- 1 tbsp. garlic powder
- Salt and black pepper to taste
- 2 tbsp. thyme, chopped
- 3 tbsp. duck fat, melted

Directions

1. Preheat Air Fryer to 380°F. In a bowl, mix duck fat, garlic powder, salt, and pepper. Add the potatoes and shake to coat.
2. Place in the basket and bake for 12 minutes, remove the basket, shake and continue cooking for another 8-

10 minutes until golden brown. Serve warm topped with thyme.

Nutrition:

Calories 110

Fat 5g

Carbs 8g

Protein 7g

Chicken Wings with Alfredo Sauce

Preparation Time: 5 minutes

Cooking time: 20 minutes

Servings: 4

Ingredients:

- 1 ½ lb. chicken wings, pat-dried
- Salt to taste
- ½ cup Alfredo sauce

Directions

1. Preheat Air Fryer to 370°F.
2. Season the wings with salt. Arrange them in the greased Air Fryer basket, without touching and Air Fry for 12 minutes until no longer pink in the center. Work in batches if needed. Flip them, increase the heat to 390°F and cook for 5 more minutes. Plate the wings and drizzle with Alfredo sauce to serve.

19

Nutrition:

Calories 150

Fat 5g

Carbs 7g

Protein 14g

Crispy Kale Chips

Preparation Time: 5 minutes

Cooking time: 10 minutes

Servings: 4

Ingredients:

- 4 cups kale leaves, stems removed, chopped
- 2 tbsp. olive oil
- 1 tsp. garlic powder
- Salt and black pepper to taste
- ¼ tsp. onion powder

Directions

1. In a bowl, mix kale and olive oil. Add in garlic and onion powders, salt, and black pepper; toss to coat.
2. Arrange the kale in the frying basket and Air Fry for 8 minutes at 350°F, shaking once. Serve cool.

Nutrition:

Calories 80

Fat 1g

Carbs 3g

Protein 3g

Crispy Squash

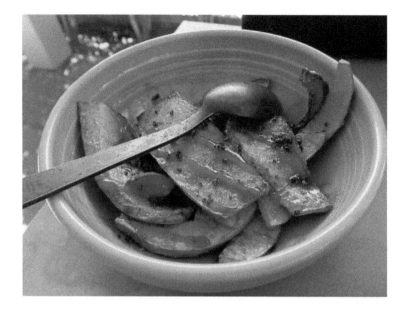

Preparation Time: 5 minutes

Cooking time: 20 minutes

Servings: 4

Ingredients:

- 2 cups butternut squash, cubed
- 2 tbsp. olive oil

- Salt and black pepper to taste
- ¼ tsp. dried thyme
- 1 tbsp. fresh parsley, finely chopped

Directions

1. In a bowl, add squash, olive oil, salt, pepper, and thyme, and toss to coat.
2. Place the squash in the Air Fryer and Air Fry for 14 minutes at 360°F, shaking once or twice. Serve sprinkled with fresh parsley.

Nutrition:

Calories 100

Fat 2g

Carbs 5g

Fat 2g

Protein 3g

Ketogenic Mac & Cheese

Preparation Time: 5 minutes

Cooking Time: 20 minutes

Servings: 4

Ingredients:

- tbsp. avocado oil
- Sea salt & black pepper to taste
- 1 cauliflower, medium
- ¼ cup heavy cream
- ¼ cup almond milk, unsweetened
- 1 cup cheddar cheese, shredded

Directions:

1. Start by preheating your Air Fryer to 400°F, and then make sure to grease your Air Fryer basket.
2. Chop your cauliflower into florets, and then Drizzle with oil over them. Toss until they're well coated, and then season with salt and pepper to taste.

25

3. Heat your cheddar, heavy cream, milk and avocado oil in a pot, pouring the mixture over your cauliflower.
4. Cook for fourteen minutes, and then serve warm.

Nutrition:

Calories 135.5

Fat 10.2g

Carbs 1.4 g

Protein 27g

Salmon Pie

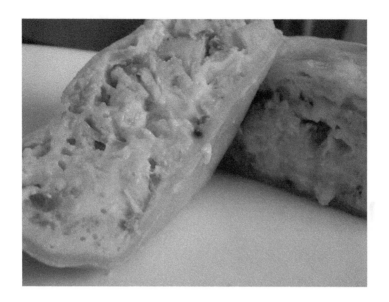

Preparation Time: 5 minutes

Cooking Time: 45 minutes

Servings: 8

Ingredients:

- 1 tsp. paprika
- ½ cup cream

27

- ½ tsp.s baking soda
- 1 ½ cups almond flour
- 1 onion, diced
- 1 tbsp. apple cider vinegar
- 1 lb. Salmon
- 1 tbsp. chives
- 1 tsp. dill
- 1 tsp. oregano
- 1 tsp. butter
- 1 tsp. parsley
- 1 egg

Directions:

1. Start by beating your eggs in a bowl, making sure they're whisked well. Add in your cream, whisking for another two minutes
2. Add in your apple cider vinegar and baking soda, stirring well.
3. Add in your almond flour, combining until it makes a non-stick, smooth dough.
4. Chop your salmon into pieces, and then sprinkle your seasoning over it.
5. Mix well, and then cut your dough into two parts.

6. Place parchment paper over your Air Fryer basket tray, placing the first part of your dough in the tray to form a crust. Add in your salmon filling.
7. Roll out the second part, covering your salmon filling. Secure the edges, and then heat your Air Fryer to 360°F.
8. Cook for 15 minutes, and then reduce the heat to 355°F, cooking for another 15 minutes
9. Slice and serve warm.

Nutrition:

Calories 134

Fat 8.1g

Carbs 2.2 g

Protein 13.2 g

Garlic Chicken Stir

Preparation Time: 5 minutes

Cooking Time: 20 minutes

Servings: 4

Ingredients:

- ½ Cup coconut milk
- ½ cup chicken stock
- tbsp. curry paste
- 1 tbsp. lemongrass
- 1 tbsp. apple cider vinegar
- tsp.s garlic, minced
- 1 onion
- 1 lb. Chicken breast, skinless & boneless
- 1 tsp. olive oil

Directions:

1. Start by cubing your chicken, and then peel your onion before dicing it.
2. Combine your onion and chicken together in your Air Fryer basket, and then preheat it to 365°F. Cook for five minutes
3. Add in your garlic, apple cider vinegar, coconut milk, lemongrass, curry paste and chicken stock. Mix well, and cook for ten minutes more.
4. Stir well before serving.

Nutrition:

Calories 275

Fat 15.7g

Carbs 5.9 g

Protein 25.6 g

Chicken Stew

Preparation Time: 5 minutes

Cooking Time: 25 minutes

Servings: 4

Ingredients:

- 1 tsp. cilantro
- oz. chicken breast, boneless & skinless
- 1 onion
- ½ cup spinach
- cups chicken stock
- oz. cabbage
- oz. cauliflower
- 1 tsp. salt
- 1 green bell pepper
- 1/3 cup heavy cream
- 1 tsp. paprika
- 1 tsp. butter
- 1 tsp. cayenne pepper

Directions:

1. Start by cubing your chicken breast, and then sprinkling your cilantro, cayenne, salt and paprika over it.
2. Heat your Air Fryer to 365°F, and then melt your butter in your Air Fryer basket.
3. Add your chicken cubes in, cooking it for 4 minutes
4. Chop your spinach, and then dice your onion.
5. Shred your cabbage and cut your cauliflower into florets. Chop your green pepper next, and then add them into your Air Fryer.
6. Pour your chicken stock and heavy cream in, and then reduce your Air Fryer to 360°F. Cook for 8 minutes, and stir before serving.

Nutrition:

Calories 102

Fat 4.5 g

Carbs 4.1 g

Protein 9.8 g

Goulash

Preparation Time: 5 minutes

Cooking Time: 12 minutes

Serving: 6

Ingredients:

- 1 white onion
- green peppers, chopped
- 1 tsp. olive oil
- 14 oz. ground chicken
- tomatoes
- ½ cup chicken stock
- 1 tsp. sea salt, fine
- cloves garlic, sliced
- 1 tsp. black pepper
- 1 tsp. mustard

Directions:

1. Peel your onion before chopping it roughly.
2. Spray your Air Fryer down with olive oil before preheating it to 365 °F.
3. Add in your chopped green pepper, cooking for five minutes
4. Add your ground chicken and cubed tomato next. Mix well, and cook for 6 minutes
5. Add in the chicken stock, salt, pepper, mustard and garlic. Mix well, and cook for 6 minutes more. Serve warm.

Nutrition:

Calories 161

Fat 6.1 g

Carbs 4.3 g

Protein 20.3 g

Beef & broccoli

Preparation Time: 5 minutes

Cooking time: 20 minutes

Servings: 4

Ingredients:

- 1 tsp. paprika
- 1 onion
- 1/3 cup water
- oz. broccoli
- oz. beef brisket
- 1 tsp. canola oil
- 1 tsp. butter
- ½ tsp. chili flakes
- 1 tbsp. flax seeds

Directions:

1. Start by chopping your beef brisket, and then sprinkle it with chili flakes and paprika. Mix your meat well, and then preheat your Air Fryer to 360°F.

2. Spray your Air Fryer down with canola oil, placing your beef in the basket tray. Cook for 7 minutes, and make sure to stir once while cooking.

3. Chop your broccoli into florets, and then add them into your Air Fryer basket next.

4. Add in your butter and flax seeds before mixing in your water. Slice your onion, adding it into it, and stir well.

5. Cook at 265°F for 6 minutes. Serve warm.

Nutrition:

Calories 187

Fat 7.3g

Carbs 3.8g

Protein 23.4g

Ground Beef Mash

Preparation Time: 5 minutes

Cooking Time: 20 minutes

Servings: 4

Ingredients:

- 1 lb. Ground beef
- 1 onion
- 1 tsp. garlic, sliced
- ¼ cup cream
- 1 tsp. white pepper
- 1 tsp. olive oil
- 1 tsp. dill
- tsp.s chicken stock
- green peppers
- 1 tsp. cayenne pepper

Directions:

1. Start by peeling your onion before grating it. Combine it with your sliced garlic, and then sprinkle your ground beef down with it. Add in your white pepper, and then add your cayenne and dill.

2. Coat your Air Fryer basket down with olive oil, heating it up to 365°F.

3. Place the spiced beef in the basket, cooking for 3 minutes before stirring. Add in the rest of your grated onion mixture and chicken stock, and then cook for 2 minutes more.

4. Chop your green peppers into small pieces, and then add them in.

5. Add in your cream, and stir well.

6. Allow it to cook for 10 minutes more.

7. Mash your mixture to make sure it's scrambled before serving warm.

Nutrition:

Calories 258

Fat 9.3g

Carbs 4.9g

Protein 35.5g

Chicken Casserole

Preparation Time: 5 minutes

Cooking Time: 30 minutes

Servings: 4

Ingredients:

- 1 tbsp. butter
- oz. round chicken
- ½ onion
- oz. bacon
- Sea salt & black pepper to taste
- 1 tsp. turmeric
- 1 tsp. paprika
- oz. cheddar cheese, shredded
- 1 egg
- ½ cup cream
- 1 tbsp. almond flour

Directions:

1. Spread your butter into your Air Fryer tray, and then add in your ground chicken. Season it with salt and pepper, and then add in your turmeric and paprika. Stir well, and then add in your cheddar cheese.

2. Beat your egg into your ground chicken, and mix well. Whisk your cream and almond flour together.

3. Peel and dice your onion, and then add it into your Air Fryer too.

4. Layer your cheese and bacon, and then heat your Air Fryer to 380°F. Cook for 18 minutes, and then allow it to cool slightly before serving.

Nutrition:

Calories 396

Fat 28.6g

Carbs 2.8g

Protein 30.4g

Chicken Hash

Preparation Time: 5 minutes

Cooking Time: 20 minutes

Servings: 3

Ingredients:

- 1 Tbsp. Water
- 1 Green Pepper
- ½ Onion
- Oz. Cauliflower
- Chicken Fillet, 7 Oz.
- 1 Tbsp. cream
- Tbsp. Butter
- Black Pepper to taste

Directions:

1. Start by roughly chopping your cauliflower before placing it in a blender. Blend until you get a cauliflower rice.

2. Chop your chicken into small pieces, and then get out your chicken fillets. Sprinkle with black pepper.

3. Heat your Air Fryer to 380°F, and then put your chicken in the Air Fryer basket. Add in your water and cream, cooking for 6 minutes

4. Reduce the heat to 360°F, and then dice your green pepper and onion.

5. Add this to your cauliflower rice, and then add in your butter. Mix well, and then add it to your chicken. Cook for 8 minutes

6. Serve warm.

Nutrition:

Calories 261

Fat 16.8g

Carbs 4.4g

Protein 21g

Pesto Tomatoes

Preparation Time: 5 minutes

Cooking Time: 10 minutes

Servings: 4

Ingredients:

- Large heirloom tomatoes – 3, cut into ½ inch thick slices.
- Pesto – 1 cup
- Feta cheese – 8 oz. cut into ½ inch thick slices
- Red onion – ½ cup, sliced thinly
- Olive oil – 1 tbsp.

Directions:

1. Spread some pesto on each slice of tomato. Top each tomato slice with a feta slice and onion and drizzle with oil. Arrange the tomatoes onto the greased rack and spray with cooking spray.

44

2. Arrange the drip pan in the bottom of the Air Fryer Oven cooking chamber. Heat at 390°F. Set the time for 14 minutes and press "Start".
3. When Cooking Time is complete, remove the rack from the Air Fryer Oven. Serve warm.

Nutrition:

Calories 480

Fat 41.9g

Carbs 13g

Protein 15.4g

Seasoned Potatoes

Preparation Time: 5 minutes

Cooking Time: 40 minutes

Servings: 2

Ingredients:

- Russet potatoes – 2, scrubbed
- Butter – ½ tbsp. melted
- Garlic & herb blend seasoning – ½ tsp.
- Garlic powder – ½ tsp.
- Salt, as required

Directions:

1. In a bowl, mix all of the spices and salt. With a fork, prick the potatoes. Coat the potatoes with butter and sprinkle with spice mixture. Arrange the potatoes onto the cooking rack. Arrange the drip pan in the bottom of the Air Fryer Oven cooking chamber.

2. Set the temperature to 400°F. Set the time for 40 minutes and press "Start." Insert the cooking rack in the center position. Once cooking is done, remove the tray from the Air Fryer Oven. Serve hot.

Nutrition:

Calories 176

Fat 2.1g

Carbs 34.2g

Protein 3.8g

Spicy Zucchini

Preparation Time: 10 minutes

Cooking Time: 15 minutes

Servings: 4

Ingredients:

- Zucchini – 1 lb. cut into ½-inch thick slices lengthwise
- Olive oil – 1 tbsp.
- Garlic powder – ½ tsp.
- Cayenne pepper – ½ tsp.
- Salt and ground black pepper, as required

Directions:

1. Put all of the ingredients into a bowl and toss to coat well. Arrange the zucchini slices onto a cooking tray. Arrange the drip pan in the bottom of the Air Fryer Oven cooking chamber.

2. Set the temperature to 400°F. Set the time for 12 minutes and press "Start." Insert the cooking tray in the center position. Once cooking is done, remove the tray from the Air Fryer Oven. Serve hot.

Nutrition:

Calories 67

Fat 5g

Carbs 5.6g

Protein 2g

Seasoned Yellow Squash

Preparation Time: 5 minutes

Cooking Time: 10 minutes

Servings: 4

Ingredients:

- Large yellow squash – 4, cut into slices
- Olive oil – ¼ cup
- Onion – ½, sliced
- Italian seasoning – ¾ tsp.
- Garlic salt – ½ tsp.
- Seasoned salt – ¼ tsp.

Directions:

1. In a bowl, mix all the ingredients together. Place the veggie mixture in the greased cooking tray. Arrange the drip pan in the bottom of the Air Fryer Oven cooking chamber.

2. Set the temperature to 400°F. Set the time for 10 minutes and press "Start". Insert the cooking tray in the center position. After 4-5 minutes turn the vegetables. Once cooking is done, remove the tray from the Air Fryer Oven. Serve hot.

Nutrition:

Calories 113

Fat 9g

Carbs 8.1g

Protein 4.2g

Buttered Asparagus

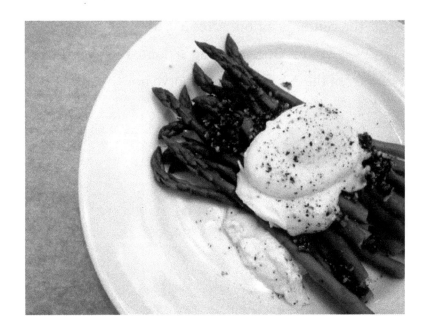

Preparation Time: 5 minutes

Cooking Time: 10 minutes

Servings: 4

Ingredients:

- Fresh thick asparagus spears – 1 lb. trimmed

- Butter – 1 tbsp. melted
- Salt and ground black pepper, as required

Directions:

1. Put all of the ingredients into a bowl and toss to coat well. Arrange the asparagus onto a cooking tray. Arrange the drip pan in the bottom of the Air Fryer Oven cooking chamber.
2. Set the temperature to 350°F. Set the time for 10 minutes and press "Start."
3. After 4-5 minutes turn the asparagus. Once cooking is done, remove the tray from Air Fryer Oven. Serve hot.

Nutrition:

Calories 64

Fat 4g

Carbs 5.9g

Protein 3.4g

Buttered Broccoli

Preparation Time: 5 minutes

Cooking Time: 15 minutes

Servings: 4

Ingredients:

- Broccoli florets – 1 lb.
- Butter – 1 tbsp. melted
- Red pepper flakes – ½ tsp. crushed
- Salt and ground black pepper, as required

Directions:

1. Gather all of the ingredients in a bowl and toss to coat well. Place the broccoli florets in the rotisserie basket and attach the lid. Arrange the drip pan in the bottom of the Air Fryer Oven cooking chamber.
2. Set the temperature to 400°F. Fix the time for 15 minutes and press "Start."
3. Arrange the rotisserie basket, on the rotisserie spit.

4. When Cooking Time is complete, remove from the Air Fryer Oven. Serve immediately.

Nutrition:

Calories 55

Fat 3g

Carbs 6.1g

Protein 2.3g

Seasoned Carrots with Green Beans

Preparation Time: 5 minutes

Cooking Time: 10 minutes

Servings: 4

Ingredients:

- Green beans – ½ lb. trimmed
- Carrots – ½ lb. peeled and cut into sticks
- Olive oil – 1 tbsp.
- Salt and ground black pepper, as required

Directions:

1. Gather all the ingredients into a bowl and toss to coat well. Place the vegetables in the rotisserie basket and attach the lid. Arrange the drip pan in the bottom of the Air Fryer Oven cooking chamber.
2. Set the temperature to 400°F. Set the time for 10 minutes and press "Start".

3. When Cooking Time is completer, emove from the
   Air Fryer Oven. Serve hot.

Nutrition:

Calories 94

Fat 4.8g

Carbs 12.7g

Protein 2g

Sweet Potato with Broccoli

Preparation Time: 5 minutes

Cooking Time: 20 minutes

Servings: 4

Ingredients:

- Medium sweet potatoes – 2, peeled and cut in 1-inch cubes
- Broccoli head – 1, cut in 1-inch florets
- Vegetable oil – 2 tbsps.
- Salt and ground black pepper, as required

Directions:

1. Grease a baking dish that will fit in the Air Fryer Oven. Gather all of the ingredients into a bowl and toss to coat well. Place the veggie mixture into the prepared baking dish in a single layer.
2. Arrange the drip pan in the bottom of the Air Fryer Oven cooking chamber. Select "Roast" and then

adjust the temperature to 415°F. Set the time for 20 minutes and press "Start".

3. Turn the vegetables every few minutes. When Cooking Time is complete, remove the baking dish from the Air Fryer Oven. Serve hot.

Nutrition:

Calories 170

Fat 7.1g

Carbs 25.2g

Protein 2.9g

Seasoned Veggies

Preparation Time: 5 minutes

Cooking Time: 12 minutes

Servings: 4

Ingredients:

- Baby carrots – 1 cup
- Broccoli florets – 1 cup
- Cauliflower florets – 1 cup
- Olive oil – 1 tbsp.
- Italian seasoning – 1 tbsp.
- Salt and ground black pepper, as required

Directions:

1. Gather all of the ingredients into a bowl and toss to coat well. Place the vegetables in the rotisserie basket and attach the lid. Arrange the drip pan in the bottom of the Air Fryer Oven cooking chamber.

2. Choose "Air Fry" and then set the temperature to 380°F. Set the time for 18 minutes and press "Start". Then, close the door and touch "Rotate".
3. When the display shows "Add Food" arrange the rotisserie basket, on the rotisserie spit. Then, close the door and touch "Rotate". When Cooking Time is complete, press the red lever to release the rod. Remove from the Air Fryer Oven. Serve.

Nutrition:

Calories 66

Fat 4.7g

Carbs 5.7g

Protein 1.4g

Potato Gratin

Preparation Time: 5 minutes

Cooking Time: 20 minutes

Servings: 4

Ingredients:

- Large potatoes – 2, sliced thinly
- Cream – 5½ tbsps.
- Eggs – 2
- Plain flour – 1 tbsp.
- Cheddar cheese – ½ cup, grated

Directions:

1. Arrange the potato cubes onto the greased rack. Arrange the drip pan in the bottom of the Air Fryer Oven cooking chamber. Choose "Air Fry" and then set the temperature to 355°F. Set the time for 10 minutes and press "Start". When the display shows "Add Food" insert the cooking rack in the center position.

2. Meanwhile, in a bowl, add cream, eggs and flour and mix until a thick sauce form. Once cooking is done, remove the tray from the Air Fryer Oven. Divide the potato slices into 4 lightly greased ramekins evenly and top with the egg mixture, followed by the cheese. Arrange the ramekins on top of a cooking rack.

3. Again, select "Air Fry" and then adjust the temperature to 390°F. Set the time for 10 minutes and press "Start". When the display shows "Add Food" insert the cooking rack in the center position. When Cooking Time is complete, remove the ramekins from the Air Fryer Oven. Serve warm.

Nutrition:

Calories 233

Fat 8g

Carbs 31.g

Protein 9.7g

Garlic Edamame

Preparation Time: 5 minutes

Cooking Time: 10 minutes

Servings: 4

Ingredients:

- Olive oil
- 1 (16 oz.) bag frozen edamame in pods
- salt and freshly ground black pepper
- ½ tsp. garlic salt
- ½ tsp. red pepper flakes (optional)

Directions:

1. Spray a fryer basket lightly with olive oil.
2. In a medium bowl, add the frozen edamame and lightly spray with olive oil. Toss to coat.
3. In a bowl, combine together the garlic salt, salt, black pepper, and red pepper flakes (if using). Add the mixture to the edamame and toss until evenly coated.

4. Place half the edamame in the fryer basket. Do not overfill the basket.

5. Air fry for 5 minutes at 360°F. Shake the basket and cook until the edamame is starting to brown and get crispy, 3 to 5 more minutes.

6. Repeat with the remaining edamame and serve immediately.

7. Pair It With: These make a nice side dish to almost any meal.

8. Air Fry Like A Pro: If you use fresh edamame, reduce the air fry time by 2 to 3 minutes to avoid overcooking. Air-fried edamame do not retain their crisp texture, so it's best to eat them right after cooking.

Nutrition:

Calories 100

Fat 3g

Carbs 9g

Protein 8g

Egg Roll Pizza Sticks

Preparation Time: 10 minutes

Cooking Time: 5 minutes

Servings: 4

Ingredients:

- Olive oil
- 8 pieces reduced-fat string cheese
- 8 egg roll wrappers
- 24 slices turkey pepperoni
- Marinara sauce, for dipping (optional)

Directions:

1. Spray a fryer basket lightly with olive oil. Fill a small bowl with water.
2. Place each egg roll wrapper diagonally on a work surface. It should look like a diamond.
3. Place 3 slices of turkey pepperoni in a vertical line down the center of the wrapper.

4. Place 1 mozzarella cheese stick on top of the turkey pepperoni.

5. Fold the top and bottom corners of the egg roll wrapper over the cheese stick.

6. Fold the left corner over the cheese stick and roll the cheese stick up to resemble a spring roll. Dip a finger in the water and seal the edge of the roll

7. Repeat with the rest of the pizza sticks.

8. Place them in the fryer basket in a single layer, making sure to leave a little space between each one. Lightly spray the pizza sticks with oil.

9. Air fry at 362°F until the pizza sticks are lightly browned and crispy, about 5 minutes.

10. These are best served hot while the cheese is melted. Accompany with a small bowl of marinara sauce, if desired.

Nutrition:

Calories 362

Fat 8g

Carbs 40g

Protein 23g

Cajun Zucchini Chips

Preparation Time: 10 minutes

Cooking Time: 15 minutes

Servings: 4

Ingredients:

- Olive oil
- 2 large zucchinis, cut into ⅛-inch-thick slices
- 2 tsp.s Cajun seasoning

Directions:

1. Spray a fryer basket lightly with olive oil.
2. Put the zucchini slices in a medium bowl and spray them generously with olive oil.
3. Sprinkle the Cajun seasoning over the zucchini and stir to make sure they are evenly coated with oil and seasoning.
4. Place slices in a single layer in the fryer basket, making sure not to overcrowd.

5. Air fry for 8 minutes at 365°F. Flip the slices over and air fry until they are as crisp and brown as you prefer, an additional 7 to 8 minutes.

6. Air Fry Like A Pro: In order to achieve the best result, it is important not to overcrowd the fryer basket. The zucchini chips turn out best if there is room for the air to circulate around each slice. You can add Cooking Time if you like very brown and crunchy zucchini chips.

Nutrition:

Calories 26

Fat <1g

Carbs 5g

Protein 2g

Crispy Old Bay Chicken Wings

Preparation Time: 10 minutes

Cooking Time: 15 minutes

Servings: 4

Ingredients:

- Olive oil
- 2 tbsp. Old Bay seasoning
- 2 tsp.s baking powder
- 2 tsp.s salt
- 2 lb. chicken wings

Directions:

1. Spray a fryer basket lightly with olive oil.
2. In a big resealable bag, combine together the Old Bay seasoning, baking powder, and salt.
3. Pat the wings dry with paper towels. Place the wings in the zip-top bag, seal, and toss with the seasoning mixture until evenly coated.

4. Place the seasoned wings in the fryer basket in a single layer. Lightly spray with olive oil.

5. Air fry for 7 minutes at 375°F. Turn the wings over, lightly spray them with olive oil, and air fry until the wings are crispy and lightly browned, 5 to 8 more minutes. Using a meat thermometer, check to make sure the internal temperature is 165°F or higher.

Nutrition:

Calories 501

Fat 36g

Carbs 1g

Protein 42g

Cinnamon and Sugar Peaches

Preparation Time: 10 minutes

Cooking Time: 13 minutes

Servings: 4

Ingredients:

- Olive oil
- 2 tbsp. sugar
- ¼ tsp. ground cinnamon
- 4 peaches, cut into wedges

Directions:

1. Spray a fryer basket lightly with olive oil.
2. In a bowl, combine the cinnamon and sugar. Add the peaches and toss to coat evenly.
3. Place the peaches in a single layer in the fryer basket on their sides.
4. Air fry for 5 minutes at 365°F. Turn the peaches skin side down, lightly spray them with oil, and air fry

until the peaches are lightly brown and caramelized, 5 to 8 more minutes.

5. Make it Even Lower Calorie: Use a zero-calorie sugar substitute such as NutraSweet or monk fruit sweetener instead of granulated sugar.

6. Air Fry Like A Pro: These do not get truly crispy, but rather they remain soft, sweet, and caramelized. They are truly delightful and make a wonderful dessert option.

Nutrition:

Calories 67

Fat <1g

Carbs 17g

Protein 1g

Chicken wings with Provencal herbs in Air Fryer

Preparation Time: 15 minutes

Cooking Time: 20 minutes

Servings: 4

Ingredients:

- 2 lb. chicken wings
- Provencal herbs
- Extra virgin olive oil
- Salt
- Ground pepper

Directions:

1. Put the chicken wings in a bowl, clean and chopped.
2. Add a few threads of oil, salt, ground pepper and sprinkle with Provencal herbs.
3. Link well and let macerate a few minutes.
4. Put the wings in the basket of the Air Fryer.

5. Select 360°F for 20 minutes.
6. From time to time remove so that they are done on all their sides
7. Serve hot

Nutrition:

Calories 160

Fat 6g

Carbs 8g

Protein 13g

Spiced Chicken wings in Air Fryer

Preparation Time: 15 minutes

Cooking Time: 30 minutes

Servings: 4

Ingredients:

- 2 lb. chicken wings
- Salt
- Ground pepper
- Extra virgin olive oil
- Spices

Directions:

1. Clean the wings and chop, throw the tip and place in a bowl the other two parts of the wings that have more meat.
2. Season and add some extra virgin olive oil threads.
3. Sprinkle with spices, put spices for roast chicken that they sell as is in supermarkets, in regular spice cans.

4. Leave for 30 minutes to rest in the refrigerator.
5. Put the wings in the basket of the Air Fryer and select 360°F, about 30 minutes. From time to time, shake the basket so that the wings move and are made all over their sides
6. Serve hot

Nutrition:

Calories 170

Fat 6g

Carbs 8g

 Protein 15g

Rosti (Swiss potatoes)

Preparation Time: 10 minutes

Cooking Time: 15 minutes

Servings: 4

Ingredients:

- 250g peeled white potatoes
- 1 tbsp. finely chopped chives
- Freshly ground black pepper
- 1 tbsp. of olive oil
- 2 tbsp. of sour cream

Directions:

1. Preheat the Air Fryer to 180°C. Grate the thick potatoes in a bowl and add three quarters of the chives and salt and pepper to taste. Mix it well.
2. Grease the pizza pan with olive oil and spread the potato mixture evenly through the pan. Press the

grated potatoes against the pan and spread the top of the potato cake with some olive oil.

3. Place the pizza pan inside the fryer basket and insert it into the Air Fryer. Set the timer to 15 mins and fry the rosti until it has a nice brownish color on the outside and is soft and well done inside.

4. Cut the rosti into 4 quarters and place each quarter on a plate. Garnish with a spoonful of sour cream. Spread the remaining of the scallions over the sour cream and add a touch of ground pepper.

Nutrition:

Calories 253g

Fat 11.7g

Carbs 25.2g

Protein 2.5g

Baked Parsley

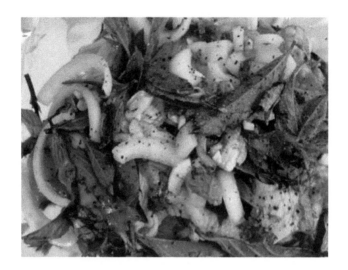

Preparation Time: 5 minutes

Cooking Time: 5 minutes

Servings: 4

Ingredients:

- 1 stick parsley
- 1 prize salt

Directions:

1. Free the fresh parsley from the coarse stalks and bake it in the Air Fryer for 5 minutes at 350°F.
2. Drain and sprinkle with a little salt.

Nutrition:

Calories 15

Fat 0g

Carbs 2g

Protein 2g

Duck thighs from the Air Fryer

Preparation Time: 5 minutes

Cooking Time: 50 minutes

Servings: 4

Ingredients:

- 2 pcs. Duck legs
- 1 tsp. salt
- 1 tsp. spice mixture (for ducks and geese)
- 1 tsp. olive oil

Directions:

1. Wash the duck legs and pat dry. Mix the oil with the salt and the spice mixture and rub the duck legs around with it.
2. Place the spiced duck legs on the hot Air Fryer's rack and cook at 400°F in 40 minutes. After 20 minutes, turn the legs once.
3. Serve hot

Nutrition:

Calories 259

Fat 28g

Carbs 0g

Protein 19g

Chopped Bondiola

Preparation Time: 5 minutes

Cooking Time: 20 minutes

Servings: 4

Ingredients:

- 2 lb. Bondiola in pieces
- Bread crumbs
- 2 eggs
- Seasoning to taste

Directions:

1. Cut the bondiola into small pieces, add seasonings to taste.
2. Whisk the eggs in a bowl
3. Pass the seasoned bondiola in the eggs and then in the breadcrumbs
4. Place it in the Air Fryer at 360°F for 20 minutes, turn after 10 minutes

5. Serve hot

Nutrition:

Calories 340

Fat 12g

Carbs 11g

 Protein 18g

Zucchini Curry

Preparation Time: 5 Minutes

Cooking Time: 8-10 Minutes

Ingredients:

- 2 Zucchinis, Washed & Sliced
- 1 Tbsp. Olive Oil
- Pinch Sea Salt
- Curry Mix, Pre-Made

Directions:

1. Turn on your Air Fryer to 390°F
2. Combine your zucchini slices, salt, oil, and spices.
3. Put the zucchini into the Air Fryer, cooking for 8 to 10 minutes.
4. You can serve alone or with sour cream.

Nutrition:

Calories 100

Fat 1g

Carbs 4g

 Protein 2g

Healthy Carrot Fries

Preparation Time: 5 Minutes

Cooking Time: 12-15 Minutes

Ingredients:

- 5 Large Carrots
- 1 Tbsp. Olive Oil
- ½ Tsp. Sea Salt

Directions:

1. Heat your Air Fryer to 390°F, and then wash and peel your carrots. Cut them in a way to form fries.
2. Combine your carrot sticks with your olive oil and salt, coating evenly.
3. Place them into the Air Fryer, cooking for twelve minutes. If they're not as crispy as you desire, then cook for 2 to 3 more minutes.
4. Serve with sour cream, ketchup or just with your favorite main dish.

Nutrition:

Calories 140

Fat 3g

Carbs 6g

Protein 7g

Simple Stuffed Potatoes

Preparation Time: 15 Minutes

Cooking Time: 35 Minutes

Ingredients:

- 4Large Potatoes, Peeled
- 2Bacon, Rashers
- ½ Brown Onion, Diced
- ¼ Cup Cheese, Grated

Directions:

1. Start by heating your Air Fryer to 350°F.
2. Cut your potatoes in half, and then brush the potatoes with oil.
3. Put it in your Air Fryer, and cook for ten minutes. Brush the potatoes with oil again and bake for another ten minutes.
4. Make a whole in the baked potato to get them ready to stuff.

5. Sauté the bacon and onion in a frying pan. You should do this over medium heat, adding cheese and stir. Remove from heat.
6. Stuff your potatoes, and cook for 4-5 minutes.

Nutrition:

Calories 180

Fat 8g

Carbs 10g

 Protein 11g

Simple Roasted Carrots

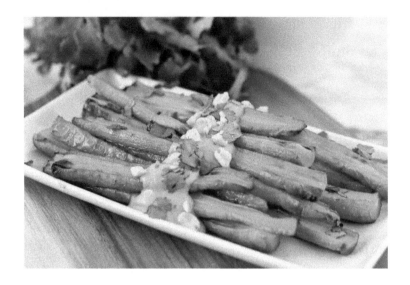

Preparation Time: 5 Minutes

Cooking Time: 35 Minutes

Ingredients:

- 4 Cups Carrots, Chopped
- 1 Tsp. Herbs de Provence
- 2 Tsp.s Olive Oil
- 4Tbsp. Orange Juice

Directions:

1. Start by preheating your Air Fryer to 320°F.
2. Combine your carrot pieces with your herbs and oil.
3. Cook for 25-28 minutes.
4. Take it out and dip the pieces in orange juice before frying for an additional 7 minutes.

Nutrition:

Calories 125

Fat 2g

Carbs 5g

Protein 6g

Broccoli & Cheese

Preparation Time: 5 Minutes

Cooking Time: 9 Minutes

Ingredients:

- 1 Head Broccoli, Washed & Chopped
- Salt & Pepper to Taste
- 1 Tbsp. Olive oil
- Sharp Cheddar Cheese, Shredded

Directions:

1. Start by putting your Air Fryer to 360°F.
2. Combine your broccoli with your olive oil and sea salt.
3. Place it in the Air Fryer, and cook for 6 minutes.
4. Take it out, and then top with cheese, cooking for another 3 minutes.
5. Serve with your choice of protein.

Nutrition:

Calories 170

Fat 5g

Carbs 9g
Protein 7g

Fried Plantains

Preparation Time: 5 minutes

Cooking Time: 10 minutes

Servings: 2

Ingredients:

- 2 ripe plantains, peeled and cut at a diagonal into ½-inch-thick pieces
- 3 tbsp. ghee, melted
- ¼ tsp. kosher salt

Directions:

1. In a bowl, mix the plantains with the ghee and salt.
2. Arrange the plantain pieces in the Air Fryer basket. Set the Air Fryer to 400°F for 8 minutes. The plantains are done when they are soft and tender on the inside, and have plenty of crisp, sweet, brown spots on the outside.

Nutrition:

Calories 180

Fat 5g

Carbs 10g

Protein 7g

Bacon-Wrapped Asparagus

Preparation Time: 5 minutes

Cooking Time: 10 minutes

Servings: 4

Ingredients:

- 1 lb. asparagus, trimmed (about 24 spears)
- 4slices bacon or beef bacon
- ½ cup Ranch Dressin for serving
- 3tbsp. chopped fresh chives, for garnish

Directions:

1. Grease the Air Fryer basket with avocado oil. Preheat the Air Fryer to 400°F.
2. Slice the bacon down the middle, making long, thin strips. Wrap 1 slice of bacon around 3 asparagus spears and secure each end with a toothpick. Repeat with the remaining bacon and asparagus.

3. Place the asparagus bundles in the Air Fryer in a single layer. (If you're using a smaller Air Fryer, cook in batches if necessary.) Cook for 8 minutes for thin stalks, 10 minutes for medium to thick stalks, or until the asparagus is slightly charred on the ends and the bacon is crispy.
4. Serve with ranch dressing and garnish with chives. Best served fresh.

Nutrition:

Calories 241

Fat 22gg

Carbs 6g

Protein 7g

Air Fried Roasted Corn on The Cob

Preparation Time: 5 minutes

Cooking Time: 10 minutes

Servings: 4

Ingredients:

- 1 tbsp. vegetable oil
- 4ears of corn
- Unsalted butter, for topping
- Salt, for topping
- Freshly ground black pepper, for topping

Directions:

1. Rub the vegetable oil onto the corn, coating it thoroughly.
2. Set the temperature of your Air Fryer to 400°F. Set the timer and grill for 5 minutes.
3. Using tongs, flip or rotate the corn.
4. Reset the timer and grill for 5 minutes more.

5. Serve with a pat of butter and a generous sprinkle of salt and pepper.

Nutrition:

Calories 265

Fat 17g

Carbs 29g

Protein 5g

Green Beans & Bacon

Preparation Time: 15 minutes

Cooking Time: 20 minutes

Servings: 4

Ingredients:

- 3 cups frozen cut green beans
- 1 medium onion, chopped
- 3 slices bacon, chopped
- ¼ cup water
- Kosher salt and black pepper

Directions:

1. In a 6 × 3-inch round heatproof pan, combine the frozen green beans, onion, bacon, and water. Toss to combine. Place the saucepan in the basket.
2. Set the Air Fryer to 375°F for 15 minutes.

3. Raise the Air Fryer temperature to 400°F for 5 minutes. Season the beans with salt and pepper to taste and toss well.
4. Remove the pan from the Air Fryer basket and cover with foil. Let it rest for 5 minutes then serve.

Nutrition:

Calories 230

Fat 10g

Carbs 14g

Protein 17g

Air Fried Honey Roasted Carrots

Preparation Time: 5 minutes

Cooking Time: 15 minutes

Servings: 4

Ingredients:

- 3cups baby carrots
- 1 tbsp. extra-virgin olive oil
- 1 tbsp. honey
- Salt
- Freshly ground black pepper
- Fresh dill (optional)

Directions:

1. In a bowl, combine honey, olive oil, carrots, salt, and pepper. Make sure that the carrots are thoroughly coated with oil. Place the carrots in the Air Fryer basket.

2. Set the temperature of your Air Fryer to 390°F. Set the timer and roast for 12 minutes, or until fork-tender.

3. Remove the Air Fryer drawer and release the Air Fryer basket. Pour the carrots into a bowl, sprinkle with dill, if desired, and serve.

Nutrition:

Calories 140

Fat 3g

Carbs 7g

Protein 9g

Air Fried Roasted Cabbage

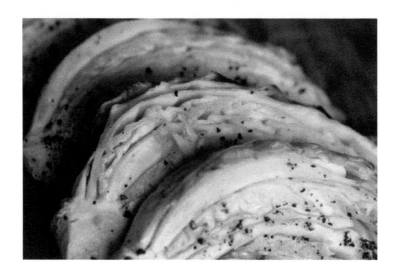

Preparation Time: 5 minutes

Cooking Time: 10 minutes

Servings: 4

Ingredients:

- 1 head cabbage, sliced in 1-inch-thick ribbons
- 1 tbsp. olive oil
- salt and freshly ground black pepper

- 1 tsp. garlic powder
- 1 tsp. red pepper flakes

Directions:

1. In a bowl, combine the olive oil, cabbage, salt, pepper, garlic powder, and red pepper flakes. Make sure that the cabbage is thoroughly coated with oil. Place the cabbage in the Air Fryer basket.
2. Set the temperature of your Air Fryer to 350°F. Set the timer and roast for 4 minutes.
3. Using tongs, flip the cabbage. Reset the timer and roast for 3 minutes more.

Nutrition:

Calories 100

Fat 1g

Carbs 3g
Protein 3g

Lightning Source UK Ltd.
Milton Keynes UK
UKHW020817170621
385664UK00001B/89